Adrenal Fatigue

Overcome Adrenal Fatigue Syndrome, Boost Energy Levels, and Reduce Stress

By Phil Smith

© **Copyright 2016 by Phil Smith. All rights reserved.**
This document is geared towards providing exact and reliable information in regards to the topic and issue covered. The publication is sold with the idea that the publisher is not required to render accounting, officially permitted, or otherwise, qualified services. If advice is necessary, legal or professional, a practiced individual in the profession should be ordered.

- From a Declaration of Principles which was accepted and approved equally by a Committee of the American Bar Association and a Committee of Publishers and Associations.

In no way is it legal to reproduce, duplicate, or transmit any part of this document in either electronic means or in printed format. Recording of this publication is strictly prohibited and any storage of this document is not allowed unless with written permission from the publisher. All rights reserved.

The information provided herein is stated to be truthful and consistent, in that any liability, in terms of inattention or otherwise, by any usage or abuse of any policies, processes, or directions contained within is the solitary and utter responsibility of the recipient reader. Under no circumstances will any legal responsibility or blame be held against the publisher for any reparation, damages, or monetary loss due to the information herein, either directly or indirectly.

Respective authors own all copyrights not held by the publisher.

The information herein is offered for informational purposes solely, and is universal as so. The presentation of the information is without contract or any type of guarantee assurance.

The trademarks that are used are without any consent, and the publication of the trademark is without permission or backing by the trademark owner. All trademarks and brands within this book are for clarifying purposes only and are the owned by the owners themselves, not affiliated with this document.

Disclaimer: This book is for informational purposes only. Use of the guidelines in this book is a choice of the reader. This book is not intended for the treatment or prevention of disease. This book is also, not a substitute for medical treatment or an alternative to medical advice.

Contents

Introduction 1

Chapter 1: What Is The Adrenal Fatigue Syndrome 2

Chapter 2: Root Causes Of Adrenal Fatigue 12

Chapter 3: Adrenal Fatigue Diagnosis 21

Chapter 4: Adrenal Fatigue Recovery 32

Chapter 5: Lifestyle Changes That Accelerate Recovery 50

Conclusion 57

Introduction

I want to thank you and congratulate you for downloading the book, Adrenal Fatigue: Overcome Adrenal Fatigue Syndrome, Boost Energy Levels, and Reduce Stress.

This book contains proven steps and strategies on how to overcome Adrenal Fatigue to live a happy and healthy life.

Do you feel overwhelmed by everyday stress? Do you find it increasingly difficult to stay in the moment? Can you remember the last time you got a good night's sleep? Do sleep with your cell phone on the charger next to your bed? Do you feel anxious but lethargic? If you answered yes to these questions, you could be suffering from adrenal fatigue syndrome and not coping with stress well. This book will explain adrenal fatigue syndrome in detail and the things you can do to recover from it.

Thanks again for downloading this book, I hope you enjoy it!

Chapter 1: What is the Adrenal Fatigue Syndrome

We have all felt overwhelmed by stress at some point in our lives. Life has a tendency of making that inevitable. It can feel like we are doing a good job of managing it, but according to our adrenal glands and hormone levels, we might actually be falling into a vicious cycle that could eventually lead to advanced adrenal fatigue syndrome. As scary as this sounds, this is actually quite common, and many people throughout the world suffer from at least one of the stages of adrenal fatigue, which we'll discuss later in this book. Even though it is still a controversial diagnosis, there are still things you can do to deal with the symptoms and recover completely.

Your adrenal glands produce hormones, one of which is cortisol. This special hormone is crucial when it comes to dealing with stress. If your adrenal glands are releasing enough cortisol, the body does not know how to deal with the stresses of daily life properly. This can lead to an array of different symptoms, one of the main ones as the name suggests is fatigue. However, the symptoms can be split up into main categories; common, which are shared by most if not all adrenal fatigue sufferers and then the more uncommon symptoms that only a handful of people suffer from. It is common for people to have a combination of both the common and uncommon symptoms.

Common Symptoms

Difficulty Getting Out of Bed

One of the most common symptoms is a difficulty getting out of bed in the morning even after getting a good night's sleep. This is especially for those who are in the earlier stages of adrenal fatigue since they are usually under intense stress. This stress is what causes the levels of cortisol and adrenaline to be too high which in turn disrupts the body's 24-hour cortisol cycle. This disruption prevents the body from getting a restful sleep because it causes a constant state of alertness.

Fatigue Each Day

In the later stages of adrenal fatigue, the body produces too little cortisol and neurotransmitters like adrenaline and norepinephrine. This means the body is not getting enough of these and the levels become too low. This explains why people with the syndrome find it difficult to maintain any energy throughout the day or to 'lift' themselves when necessary. There is an exception though which will be explained later because some sufferers find they have an increase in energy later in the day.

Stress

Those who are in the later stages have a difficult time handling stress for the same reason as the tiredness. When the body encounters stress, we rely on the adrenal gland to produce enough cortisol, adrenaline, and norepinephrine to increase our alertness, strength and focus when we need it most. If our body does not produce this when we need it to, in the correct amounts, our bodies will not respond appropriately. This leads to feelings of disinterest, apathy, anxiety, and even irritability, all of which are common amongst those in the later stages of the syndrome.

Salty Food Cravings

The cortex, a part of the adrenals, is responsible for producing a mineralocorticoid called aldosterone which works with the kidneys to regulate mineral and fluid excretions. When the adrenals are fatigued, not enough aldosterone is produced, and many important minerals are flushed out through urination. This means that many adrenal fatigue sufferers are often unable to balance the levels of minerals such as potassium, magnesium, and sodium in their blood. The body will begin to search for a way to replace the missing minerals, such as craving salty foods to replace the sodium the body lost.

Energy Late in the Day

Cortisol levels are supposed to be at their highest in the morning and then slowly declining throughout the day. However, someone in the early stages of the syndrome, when the adrenals are still capable of producing higher levels of the chemicals, can find an increase in energy later in the day because of an increase in cortisol. So if you find yourself with a strange surge of energy when you have been sluggish all day, this could be a good indicator of why.

Weakened Immune System

Cortisol also helps reduce unnecessary inflammation in the body which helps to regulate the immune system. Inflammation is generally just a symptom of the body healing or fighting an infection and cortisol helps keep it from getting out of control. That is why having balanced cortisol levels is so important. If stress is causing your cortisol levels to be too high, then the anti-inflammatory effect is too strong and prevents the immune system from acting as it should. This weakened state can last as long as the stress that caused it. On the other hand, if your cortisol levels are too low, the body can overreact and cause chronic inflammation or some auto-immune diseases.

Other Uncommon Symptoms

- Joint pain
- Dizziness
- Dark circles under the eyes
- Asthma
- Weight gain
- Loss of muscle
- Low sex drive
- Dry skin
- Low blood sugar
- Low blood pressure

You do not need to suffer from the entire list of symptoms to suffer from adrenal fatigue, as a matter of fact, most people don't. Depending on which stage of the syndrome you are currently in and other health factors such as your age, weight, and diet can determine which symptoms are more prevalent and worrisome than others. It is a good idea to keep a list of your symptoms, so you are prepared when you go the doctor. It is easy to forget something important when face to face with your doctor, but if you are armed with a pre-made list, you will be more prepared to explain your symptoms and ask the questions you want the answers to. Just the act of being and feeling prepared can also help to reduce stress.

Four main stages mark the path to adrenal fatigue that the body goes through. It is possible to overcome these stages on our own and even go in and out of them throughout our lifetimes. Their symptoms become more powerful and more prevalent as the body continues towards stage four, which is the hardest to overcome. Each stage is characterized by the different things the body goes through, beginning with the alarm phase and eventually ending with a burnout. Your doctor or naturopath will go over your specific symptoms and lab work to determine which stage you have reached and decide what an appropriate form of treatment would be.

4 Stages of Adrenal Fatigue

Stage 1 - Alarm

The first stage is known as the alarm phase; this is the body's immediate reaction to a stressor. This stressor can be anything from a hospital stay, test, or an immediate physical threat. It is during this stage of the stress reaction that the body begins to produce high levels of adrenaline, norepinephrine, insulin, DHEA, and cortisol. These are all the chemicals needed by the body to prepare the correct response to the stressor. Since the body is still capable of producing high levels of these chemicals most people in this stage have a raised sense of arousal and alertness, both of which often interrupt a healthy sleep cycle.

Many people do not report symptoms during this stage, and it is possible to go in and out of this stage throughout our lives. There is usually no physical or physiological dysfunction that can be noted clinically during this stage. Normal daily function is also common. However, peak performance is generally not achieved.

Stage 2 – Continued Alarm

The second stage is the continuation of the alarm stage; it is during this stage that the stress response continues along with the body's reaction to it. During the second stage, the endocrine system is still able to produce the hormones you need, but levels of sex hormones such as DHEA could start to decline rapidly. This happens because the resources needed to produce the sex hormones are being rerouted to the production of necessary stress hormones like cortisol.

It is also during this stage that you will begin to feel the effects of the over-worked adrenals. It is often described as the "wired … but tired" feeling. This is when some sufferers become dependent on coffee or caffeine. Our bodies can maintain alertness during the day, but they crash hard during the evening. Normal daily function can also be achieved during this stage, but you will start to notice that the body needs more rest to recover. PMS and menstrual irregularities can also begin during this stage. Other symptoms that often suggest hypothyroidism also surface, such as a feeling of coldness or a slower metabolism.

Stage 3 - Resistance

During this stage your body will still produce stress hormones at the expense of sex hormones, causing even more of a drop in sex drive. There will be substantial drops in hormones like testosterone and DHEA because hormone precursor material is sent to continue its production of the stress hormones like cortisol. The determining hormone here is called pregnenolone and which is the forerunner of both sex hormones and cortisol and when it is diverted it is called the 'pregnenolone steal.' Sufferers during this stage can still hold down a job and live a relatively normal life. However, the low hormone levels can significantly reduce their quality of life. Common symptoms during this stage can be low sex drive, regular tiredness, regular infections, and a general lack of enthusiasm. Toxic metabolites build up in the body which can lead to brain fog and insomnia. This stage can last months or even years.

Stage 4 - Burnout

After some time, the body simply runs out of ways to consistently produce stress hormones, and cortisol levels begin to decline. This means that the levels of both stress and sex hormones are too low. This leads to the burnout, or what happens to our bodies after coping with stress, as it is almost as if the body is giving up. Symptoms during this phase include lack of sex drive, weight loss, irritability, depression, apathy, anxiety, and a general disinterest in the surrounding world. The low hormone levels have an impact on almost every part of the body. It is often during this stage that sufferers find it difficult to hold down a job and it becomes increasingly to lead a normal life. Stage four can feel so powerful and overwhelming that to overcome it; a complete lifestyle change is often necessary.

Most adrenal fatigue sufferers rarely make it stage three or four and recover during the first two. That is why it is important to know which stage you are in so you know what can be done to help you overcome it before it progresses to the next stage. Stage three is considered the terminal stage of the process since it is during this stage that the body switches to focus on the conservation of energy just to ensure survival. What separates stages two and three is that during stage three you are not able to function throughout the day smoothly no matter how much effort you put forth. It is also during this stage that the smallest stressor can cause an adrenal crash.

During the fourth stage, adrenal crisis may begin to happen which can include lower back pain, dehydration, vomiting, and diarrhea. Some people will seek medical help before an adrenal crisis hits, but others choose to wait until the problem persists and these new symptoms force them to. Try to seek out the help of a doctor or naturopath before it progresses this far. Once it gets to this stage, it is increasingly difficult to treat and takes much longer to achieve a full recovery.

It doesn't matter which stage you have reached of adrenal fatigue; there are still things that can be done to help you overcome it. The journey to recovery might not be easy or happen overnight, but it is possible. Just remember, there is no one right answer when it comes to overcoming adrenal fatigue, but understanding which stages you are in will increase your chances of a full recovery.

Chapter 2: Root Causes of Adrenal Fatigue

Adrenal fatigue has been around for as long as we have, but it is only within the last 100 years that it has been considered a silent epidemic. One of the reasons that it has become more of an issue throughout this time is because of how much our lifestyles have changed.

Today our stress levels, toxic load, and diet is much worse than it was at the start of the twentieth century. It might seem like technology is making our lives easier and taking us forward, but it is actually one of the reasons we are more bogged down by stress. Our phones and tablets make it all the more difficult to just get away for a few minutes a day. There is almost always something we could be doing on our phone instead of just being in the moment, such as playing a game or returning a text. We also have the means to streamline food production, which has added even more chemicals to the prepackaged meals we eat, things our body did not evolve consuming. So, while it might feel like a good thing, it is more like a double-edged sword.

The most basic cause of adrenal fatigue is the failure of your adrenal glands to cope with stress. When determining the cause of adrenal fatigue, some factors need to be taken into consideration, such as the timeline. Adrenal fatigue does not happen overnight; it usually takes years to develop to the last two stages. So when determining what type of stressor it was that triggered your pathway to adrenal fatigue, it is important to think about past stressors. Of the basic stressors that cause adrenal fatigue, it can be a combination of many that act as a trigger or just one. The reality is that it can be difficult to figure out exactly which traumatic, stressful event triggered the downward spiral.

Even though it might be important to you to figure out what the initial trigger or triggers were that made this happen, it is healthier to look towards the future. Instead of dwelling on the past, think about how you can cope with stress in the future once you are on the road to recovery. It is okay to look at the past and learn from your mistakes, but worrying about it all the time is only going to cause you more stress.

Root Causes

Emotional Stress

It is known that stress is the most common cause of adrenal fatigue. Stress can creep up on you, stressors that feel like they are manageable in the short-term can have negative long-term consequences on your health. Stress such as looking after a newborn baby, relocating for a new job, a bad romantic relationship, or even taking an important test are all examples of emotional stressors that can lead to adrenal fatigue in the long run.

Emotional stressors are the things we face during our daily lives, the things we are forced to cope with. Even though we think we are being successful at coping, our bodies might not feel the same way, triggering the beginning of adrenal fatigue. This can happen because we stay in the situation that is causing the stress, such as the bad relationship or the stressful job for too long, prolonging the stress response and our body's reaction to it. Emotional stress has a tendency to snowball and what once seemed like a couple of small stressors can suddenly feel like a mountain resting on your shoulders.

Diet

We eat worse now than we ever have before. More and more of our diets are made up of prepackaged, processed foods and a shift away from fresh produce and vegetables. This is because we have the technology to do so and it is more convenient to eat this way. Today the average American consumes about 150 pounds of sugar per year, while 200 years ago it was only 1 or 2 pounds. Our genetics did not change in that amount of time, so our bodies had to learn to deal with a dramatic increase. Our bodies cope with the extra empty calories by creating extra insulin and cortisol which puts stress on the pancreas and adrenals.

Being overweight can also put stress on the adrenals, and one of the reasons people gain weight is eating too many calories. This is an obvious connection, but not many people relate it to adrenal fatigue. Just think of it like this, if being overweight makes you feel tired, it is probably tiring out your adrenals too. Being overweight can also cause depression and anxiety, both of which can cause more stress.

Lack of Sleep

We have all felt spread too thin at some point in our lives like we are burning the candle at both ends. We often struggle to find a work-life balance, like there are just not enough hours in the day to get everything done that needs to be done. Chances are, if you feel like this, you aren't getting enough sleep. Our ancestors had a healthy 9 hours of sleep per night, but many of us survive on less than half that. The average American sleeps 6.1 hours per night, and those even in the early stages of adrenal fatigue can get much less than that.

Sleep is how the body repairs itself and recovers from the stressors of the day. It's amazing how the body is capable of healing itself, but it still needs time to do so. Not getting enough sleep denies our body the time it needs to heal and recover properly. Getting the recommended 7 or 8 hours of sleep encourages the adrenal glands to continue to function properly.

Pollutants and Chemicals

Pollutants and chemicals are toxic loads, the general level of toxicity that we are faced with in our daily lives. Examples of this are pesticides on our foods, chlorine in our drinking water, antibiotics in our meat, and pollutants in our air. Each year 2,000 new chemicals are introduced to the consumer marketplace, many of which are never tested for human safety. Some of these chemicals are put into the food we eat and the products we buy, which can accumulate in our bodies and compromise our immune system and even lead to heart disease or even Alzheimer's.

Many of these chemicals are known to affect the adrenals directly. Our bodies are capable of making short-term adjustments to compensate, but over time the stress placed on adrenal function will take its toll leading to adrenal fatigue.

Chronic Disease

Long-term stressors to the adrenals can also include chronic diseases. It doesn't matter what type of chronic illness it is, asthma, arthritis, diabetes, and any other can place demands or impact your adrenal glands in a way that is considered above the norm. When you suffer from a chronic illness for a long period, your adrenals can become over-worked. Treatment for chronic illness is also taxing on the body, which in turn can place extra strain on the adrenals. The combination of the disease itself and the treatment can act as the trigger and catalyst for adrenal fatigue.

Trauma

Long-term factors are not the only things that can trigger adrenal fatigue. Sometimes all it takes is moments of severe physical trauma. We used to think that one moment of severe trauma would not have a long-lasting impact on our body aside from the scars and the healing time. However, we now know that is not the case, evidence suggests that these moments can have many negative long-term effects that can include hormonal balance and adrenal performance. It is not just major accidents that fall into this category; major surgeries can also cause the same long-term disruptions within the body. If you think it was a severe trauma that led to adrenal fatigue look back in your personal history and consider both major accidents and surgeries since both can have a major impact on the body.

This list breaks down the possible causes of adrenal fatigue into categories, but it is difficult to fully comprehend how much we come into contact with them until you think about how we live today. Just look at how much our lives have changed in the last 50 years. In the 1950's and 1960's, it was possible to get a good paying job without the added stress of higher education. That is not the case today. To gain a competitive advantage and get a good job it is almost necessary to go to college. Then after college, finding a job, and paying for what is now a very expensive education can all be very stressful and overwhelming. As you've learned, even if you think you are coping well, it does not mean your body is. These stressors can all add up and eventually take a toll on adrenal function.

Herein lies the problem, these stressors are hidden in the necessities we need to live, from the foods we eat to the air we breathe. Just getting a job is ridden with potential stressors that can negatively impact our bodies, sometimes to the point of adrenal fatigue. Fifty years ago it was possible for one income to pay the mortgage and it was possible to separate work life and home life. Fast forward to today and that no longer applies. Now it usually takes two incomes to pay student loans and mortgages, with both parties working longer hours than our parents or grandparents.

We have also created a consumer society which also adds to already mounting financial burdens. We are often focused on keeping up with trends and purchasing the newest and best products. We are also guilty of not being able to separate home and work, and the line becomes blurred with every work email we send late at night or every conference call we take before we even arrive at work. Our general way of living has changed to the point of having very little in common with Americans 50 years ago.

As you can see it becomes nearly impossible to hide from stress, it is all around us. That means it is even more difficult to decide what it was that triggered the adrenal fatigue in the first place. As we become busier and our lives become more hectic, we receive even less sleep. It can become a vicious cycle and very difficult to get out of. We have a distraction and added stress at our fingertips now, with the invention of computers and smartphones. This is just another one of the many examples of how we can't escape the stresses of our lives.

In addition to all the real life stressors we face, as humans we also have a tendency to imagine stressors too, it could be something that could happen, a what if situation. Even though this is a perceived stressor, our brain still treats it as though it is real and it too can trigger the stress response. A good example of this is when you have a big test to take, the amount of studying you do is stressful, hoping you don't forget anything is stressful. These both make sense because you did a study for the test and you do need to remember information to pass it. However, right before you fall asleep, you worry about oversleeping and missing the test. This is an imagined stressor; it is something that has not happened but still, causes you stress that your body is going to be forced to cope with.

Chapter 3: Adrenal Fatigue Diagnosis

Diagnosing adrenal fatigue from a single lab test or symptom is impossible. To make an accurate diagnosis doctors or naturopaths must take note of every symptom and run many tests sometimes multiple times to make the necessary comparisons. People often visit their doctors sometimes before they receive a diagnosis of adrenal fatigue. A diagnosis of adrenal fatigue is also a controversial one since so many doctors do not acknowledge it as a problem. It is for this reason that you need to be patient if you are searching for a definitive diagnosis from a doctor.

Many tests are run when diagnosing adrenal fatigue, such as the standard hormone tests that check the levels of thyroid hormones including cortisol. Then there are tests used by more integrative naturopaths and doctors which look for neurotransmitters and other various hormones that give a more accurate understanding of how the patient is feeling. It is also important that your doctor gets direct feedback from you as well. Since many tests will likely come back within range, it is important they speak with you to gain a full understanding of your symptoms. This will also give you a better chance of getting a correct diagnosis and knowing which stage you're at.

Tests

Cortisol

As you probably guessed, the major lab test to determine adrenal fatigue checks cortisol levels. Doctors can do this using blood, urine, and saliva samples. It is thought that saliva provides the best results because it gives the better estimate of the cortisol level in your cells where the hormone reactions take place. It is important to drink water before your test because of dehydration and skew the results. Taking a single measurement of cortisol levels is not enough, your doctor should request tests taken throughout the day to compare during your 24-hour cortisol cycle. This is important because our cortisol levels are highest in the mornings and decline throughout the day. Your doctor needs to know how much yours is declining and whether there is a spike later in the day.

It is also important to find a doctor who has experience with adrenal fatigue since interpreting the results is as important as the tests themselves. This can be very difficult for a doctor who does not have previous experience with adrenal fatigue. The reference ranges for labs are so wide that only abnormally low levels are given special attention. So your doctor will need to look at the different results to make his or her own judgment. It is for this reason that it is important to use the optimal range rather than a reference range.

ACTH Challenge

This is another test your doctor might run to check your cortisol levels. Your baseline cortisol levels are tested first and then you are given a shot of adrenal corticotrophic hormone. This will stimulate your adrenal hormone output which is similar to what would happen if you were facing a stressful situation. This test allows your doctor to see how your adrenals react to stress. If your cortisol shows a spike that is at least double than the initial test, then your adrenals are probably functioning properly. If the spike is not at least double, it could suggest an adrenal insufficiency.

Thyroid Tests

The complexity of the human body means that one part of the endocrine system cannot function independently of another part. There are connections in the human body between every system, and weakness in one area and lead to changes and insufficiencies in another. When dealing with adrenal fatigue evidence shows that a weakening in the pituitary gland and the hypothalamus can be a precursor to lower thyroid function. If your blood tests come back and they show mild hypothyroidism as the culprit, the underlying issue could still be adrenal fatigue.

There are many different tests used to check thyroid function, all of them are blood tests, and when your doctor interprets the results, he or she should look for more than just the recommended reference ranges.

TSH

The hypothalamus instructs the pituitary gland to produce thyroid stimulating hormone. Just as the name suggests, this hormone then tells the thyroid to produce T3 and T4 which are two most important thyroid hormones. The level of TSH is inversely proportional to thyroid activity. So if your thyroid is producing a lot of T3 and T4 the thyroid will pump out less TSH, because of the thyroid less stimulation. On the other hand, if you are hypothyroid then your TSH is likely to be high since your brain is signaling the thyroid to produce more hormones. Cortisol has a similar feedback loop, just like many other hormones present in the body.

People who suffer from adrenal fatigue often have a thyroid that is not performing well so their TSH reading might be above 2.0. The reference range in the lab is generally around 0.50 – 4.50, so you see the importance of checking optimal levels instead of just the reference ranges. Even though it falls within the range, a problem could still exist, your doctor should take this into consideration.

Free T3/T4

The free T3 test is only performed on hyperthyroid patients, but it can provide useful information into the overall function of the thyroid. It should be used in conjunction with the other thyroid tests because it can help to provide a complete image of why the thyroid is not performing properly.

Similar to the free T3 test, the free T4 test is also rarely performed, especially since T4 generally has less of an effect on the body. When your thyroid does not produce enough T4, your TSH will be higher. This blood test specifically checks for 'unbound' T4 that is available for immediate use.

Total Thyroxine

This test should be used in conjunction with the free T4 test because it also includes the T4 that is bound to carrier proteins. That means that using this test with the free T4 test will tell your doctor how much T4 is both available for use and how much is held in reserve.

Cortisol/DHEA Ratio

This test can tell your doctor which stage of adrenal fatigue you have reached. During the first stages of a stress reaction both DHEA and cortisol will be high, but as the body struggles to produce enough stress hormones, DHEA levels will begin to drop. This test shows whether or not the 'pregnenolone steal' is happening. Further on in the development of adrenal fatigue cortisol levels begin to decline as the body exhausts all capabilities of production. This ratio, in combination with other tests and information, can help your doctor determine which stage of adrenal fatigue the patient has entered.

17-Hp/Cortisol Ratio

17-hyroxyprogesterone is the raw material that the body uses to create cortisol. Adrenal fatigue sufferers typically see higher levels of 17-HP compared to cortisol because the body struggles to make the conversion happen as it should.

In addition to the tests above, there are other tests that doctors typically use to help determine if adrenal fatigue is the correct diagnosis. These are not tests that are sent to labs and are not as accurate as blood, saliva, or urine tests, but they are helpful when used in combinations with other tests. The results of these tests will help your doctor get an idea of your overall health.

Postural Low Blood Pressure

For those who are in good health when they stand, they experience an immediate increase in blood pressure. However, those with adrenal fatigue will see no change in blood pressure or even a slight drop. The more drastic the drop, the more severe case of adrenal fatigue.

Iris Contraction

This test measures the contraction of the iris when repeatedly exposed to dark light. It is thought that a weakened adrenal function means that the iris will not be able to maintain the contraction for very long.

Despite the fact that adrenal fatigue is getting more and more common and that tests can suggest to the very issue, many doctors are still not willing to diagnose it. One of the reasons doctors are so hesitant to give the diagnosis of adrenal fatigue is because lab tests can be inconclusive. There are amazingly wide ranges that labs use as their acceptable reference ranges. They look at a cross-section of the population, measure their cortisol levels, and based on this information set their reference range at two standard deviations from the mean.

As you already know, the best way to test cortisol is to check it at multiple times throughout the day. It is natural for our cortisol levels to fluctuate within a 24 hour period and to get an understanding of your specific fluctuation, more than one test is needed. These are the acceptable cortisol ranges from Labcorp:

Morning: 0.025 - 0.60 mcg/dL

Noon: 0.01 - 0.33 mcg/dL

Afternoon: 0.01 - 0.20 mcg/dL

Evening: 0.01 - 0.09 mcg/dL

As you can see, this is an incredibly wide reference range, since it is saying that you could have a noon measurement of 0.01 and be within range, but so would a measurement of 0.33, even though it is 33 times higher. In other words, your cortisol level could fall from 0.33 to 0.01, which is a staggering 97% drop, but technically you would still be within the reference range. This is why a good naturopath or doctor will use an optimal range rather than one provided by the lab. You should also note that men and women could have different optimal and reference ranges, so if you are researching on your own make sure to specify.

Wide ranges make it more difficult for doctors to appropriately treat and even diagnose their patients. There is a lot of pressure on doctors to not to 'overprescribe' drugs, making it difficult for them to justify prescribing cortisol to a patient whose levels are technically within range. Many doctors just do not feel comfortable going against what the lab is telling them. However, there are some doctors out there who do think adrenal fatigue is a valid diagnosis, so make sure that during your first visit you ask, this saves both of you time and money.

Doctors often refer to checklists (as guidelines) when diagnosing the stages of adrenal fatigue. They can compare them to previous visits to see if the symptoms are worsening or remaining the same. It is important your doctor listens to you about your specific symptoms because it isn't until the later stages that the results will reflect it and it is much easier to recover if you have not yet reached the later stages. If your doctor catches it early enough, you can look forward to a faster, easier recovery.

Insurance companies and commercial pressures also discourage doctors from diagnosing adrenal fatigue. Each disease that is recognized by insurance companies has a code, or International Classifications of Disease code, which is made and given out by the World Health Organization. There is no code for adrenal fatigue. Theoretically, doctors could use the code for adrenocortical insufficiency not otherwise specified, but in practice, this would prove very challenging because most lab tests would come back within range.

This might seem like more of a bureaucratic issue than a real problem, but without a code, doctors are unable to bill insurance companies. This means that if they diagnose you with adrenal fatigue they are not going to get paid for treating you, and we all know that doctors are not free. It can be difficult to find a more open-minded doctor. Another incentive doctors have for avoiding an adrenal fatigue diagnosis is that it is difficult to treat. A good treatment often involves herbal supplements and dietary changes, sometimes even hormone replacement. The symptoms are often easier to treat than the underlying cause and more profitable for the doctor as well.

Another option that you have is just to accept that you will be paying for all the costs associated with adrenal fatigue out of pocket. Due to all the lab work, tests, and visits, it is going to get very expensive fast. If you have the money, finding a doctor who is willing to give adrenal fatigue as a diagnosis might be easier because you are not dealing with the insurance company at all. So if this is an option for you, consider calling around until you find a doctor that has experience with someone who has suffered from adrenal fatigue. On the other hand, if you choose to forego a doctor altogether and choose to go to naturopath you will most likely be paying out of pocket too. It is also important, to be honest, and upfront with your naturopath about your symptoms. Whether you choose to go to a doctor or a naturopath or a doctor is your personal preference. They would probably ask similar questions and give you very similar advice in the end since the best way to recover from adrenal fatigue is a more natural approach.

The medical world's inability to see varying degrees is nothing new. For instance, Addison's disease is a severe adrenal insufficiency, and it is an accepted diagnosis in the medical community. However, mild adrenal insufficiency or adrenal fatigue is considered an invalid diagnosis. A few years ago endocrinologists were hesitant to diagnose hypothyroidism if a patient's tests came back within the accepted ranges, but now they will diagnose mild hypothyroidism if their tests come back on the lower end. This evolution took nearly 20 years, but we will hopefully see the same thing with adrenal fatigue.

Chapter 4: Adrenal Fatigue Recovery

It is estimated that nearly 80% of people in the world suffer from adrenal fatigue. Most people struggle with adrenal fatigue at some point during their lives, whether it be short or long-term. This means that very few of us are safe from the stresses of our daily lives. However, there are things you can do to begin your journey to recovery. In general, treatment for adrenal fatigue involves reducing stress on both the body and mind, increasing positive thinking, and replenishing your body with healthy foods and eliminating toxins.

Adrenal fatigue took a while to take hold of you, so it is safe to assume you are not going to be able to get rid of it overnight. On the other hand, it will not take as long to recover as it did for adrenal fatigue to set in. Our bodies are capable of doing incredible things, and one of them is healing. Our body can heal itself from the inside out if given the right essential building blocks. A big part of recovery is making sure you are setting the body up for the things it needs to start and continue the healing process. Once you begin to feel better, this will serve as a great motivator for success. When your energy levels start to improve, and you feel like you got a good night's rest, you will start to think that all the hard work and changes are worth it.

There is no magic cure for adrenal fatigue, and one of the most important things to remember is to be patient with yourself. It seems like there is no light at the end of the tunnel, but there can be if you keep an open mind and make changes as you see fit. This can include giving up things you have come to depend on or incorporating an exercise routine. Your success greatly depends on your dedication and effort. You can make your recovery work for you, cater to your strengths and weaknesses and when you find something that works, stick with it.

A Guideline for Recovery

Sleep

We know that one of the first symptoms of adrenal fatigue is an inability to feel rested even after a long night of rest. In the later stages, insomnia is even common. One of the best things you can do to fight adrenal fatigue is to get the recommended amount of sleep per night. First, you need to set up a routine or a pattern, give yourself a bedtime or at least a lights out time that you can stick to. Turn your bedroom into an electronic stimulus-free zone, if you have a television in your room, remove it. Now there are hundreds of channels to choose from, and it is incredibly easy to stay up all night in an entertainment loop.

This also goes for the smartphones and tablets as well. The beep or ding from a phone indicating a text message or a notification is a temptation that is easily given into when we should be sleeping. Turning off your phone at night might seem difficult, but it is necessary if you want to sleep well. If for some reason you don't want to turn it off, do not bring it in your bedroom to charge. Keep your bedroom electronic stimulus-free and charge it another room and change the settings to only allow emergency calls through.

Turn off all devices at least half an hour before bed. Evidence shows that using screens before bed suppresses the body's production of the hormone melatonin. This hormone is important because it helps us to maintain a Circadian rhythm, which is why it is often referred to as the sleep hormone. If your devices are not turned off in time, your melatonin levels might be disturbed. Also, do not get up in the middle of the night to check your different devices, this is a bad habit to get into. The exposure to the bright screen, even for a short period can prevent you from going back to sleep.

It is important if you focus on creating a relaxing environment. Another way to do this is to eliminate sources of light. Our brains are sensitive, and it is possible for even the most unassuming things to prevent it from shutting down for the night. Look around your room at night and see what other sources of light you can remove, this could mean shutting down appliances to investing in blackout curtains. A sleep mask is also a good option.

Make yourself as comfortable as possible, stop settling for the uncomfortable bedding you have. It is important to consider everything from the firmness of your mattress to the material your sheets are made from. Find what works for you and makes you the most comfortable. Adjust the temperature in your room; some people prefer a colder room while others like it to be warmer. It is personal preference and all about finding your ideal combination. If you do not have a lot of money to spend on a new mattress purchase a mattress pad or a memory foam topper. Add or take away pillows until you find the perfect, comfortable sleeping combination. If you sleep with a partner, talk to them about what you are doing and see what they do to make your night's sleep better.

It is also important to reduce noise in your room. You can do this by making sure all your devices are switched off and closing your windows to block out external noise. Some people prefer to invest some soft, comfortable ear plugs. If there are some noises that you can't block out, like snoring, for instance, purchasing a white noise machine could help. These little machines mimic the sounds of rain, waterfalls, or even ceiling fans. Some people like to put a box fan in their room that they turn on during their nightly ritual, the sound can also help let the body know that it is time to sleep.

It is also important to do things during the say that promote a good night's sleep such as exercising and a bedtime routine. All forms of exercise expend energy which will help you sleep through the night. If you set up a habitual bedtime routine, your body will come to recognize the actions as a prelude to going bed, sending the signal to your body that is it is time to sleep. An example of a bedtime routine would be checking all the doors, brushing your teeth, kissing your partner goodnight and then crawling into bed. It doesn't need to be anything elaborate, just something that you do every night, which becomes a habit. This, with the combination of regular exercise, can make a difference in an irregular sleeping pattern.

During the day try to expose yourself to some natural light. Getting a good night's sleep is about the balance between light and dark to maintain a natural rhythm. It only takes about an hour of natural sunlight to act a synchronizer for your daily hormone cycles. You should aim for bright light during the day and total darkness at night. This is why blackout curtains and reducing unnecessary light is so important to the sleep cycle; it can help to find that balance.

Diet

The food you eat is crucial because it serves as your first line of defense against adrenal fatigue. When creating an adrenal-supportive diet, there are two aspects that need to be looked at: foods that will make adrenal fatigue worse and foods that will aid your recovery. It is also important to eat meals at the right times and to consume lots of whole foods. This is not a strict diet, but it does consist of eating more fruits and vegetables and avoiding foods that are known to cause inflammation.

It is crucial that you avoid foods you know you have even a slight allergy or sensitivity to. Food intolerances and sensitivities prevent our bodies from absorbing and the using the nutrients we need. This can also lead to inflammation which can then, in turn, interfere with our sleep/wake cycle. If we are unable to absorb all the nutrients in our food, we can be left weakened and without energy. If you have any food allergies or sensitivities, it is a good idea to just cut them out of your diet altogether.

Breakfast is the most important meal of the day, and this could not be truer than when it comes to adrenal fatigue. When we sit down for breakfast, we have been fasting for the past 12 hours. Food is the way we refuel, and after fasting for 12 hours we need to do it right. The food we eat needs to supply us with enough energy to get through the morning. Your breakfast should consist of a high-quality protein and a few high-quality carbohydrates. A good example of this would be two poached eggs with blueberries or a vegetable omelet. A typical American breakfast full of sugar such as cereals or waffles is exactly what you should be avoiding. In general, if it is prepackaged, it is a safe bet to avoid it.

Many people like to prepare their meals ahead of time because it saves them time and the stress of planning out dinner at the last minute. This can also save you money and time throughout the week. You might have to give up some of your favorite junk foods, but you might find something you like even better that is also healthy. Be adventurous with your cooking and meal plans, feel free to experiment with colorful fruits and vegetables. Remember, fruits still contain sugar, so moderation is key.

It is common for adrenal fatigue sufferers to struggle with maintaining blood sugar levels during the day. This is because cortisol is closely involved with blood sugar stability. To combat this adrenal fatigue sufferers should eat many small meals throughout the day, with a maximum of three intervals. Doing this can also help reduce food cravings, and blood sugar crashes as well.

Eat less sugar, excess sugar needs to be controlled by cortisol and by eating too much of it you are indirectly taxing your adrenal glands. The crash that inevitably follows a spike in blood sugar leads to sugar cravings, and for many also the use of stimulants like caffeine to counteract the fatigue. Sugar is lurking in more things than just cakes and cookies; it can also be found in things that seem healthy such as fruit juices. Beans, sprouted grains, and vegetables are better carbohydrate options. Eating enough protein is a great way to maintain energy levels without causing spikes in your blood sugar. Free-range chicken, wild fish, beef, and eggs are all good sources of protein. If possible try to buy organic, since there are fewer additives and hormones used, these are often cheaper at your local farmer's market. Coconut, seeds, butter, cheese, and dairy are all acceptable sources of healthy fats, just make sure they are from natural, whole foods.

Making sure you stay hydrated is important no matter who you are, so make sure you are drinking water throughout the day. In addition to the more traditional foods mentioned above, there are other foods that are not part of a regular Western diet that can help you recover more quickly. One of these is bone broth. This is based on how our ancestors utilized every part of the animal, including the bone marrow which is full of valuable nutrition. Bone broth helps to reduce inflammation, encourage healthy cholesterol, and boost the immune system, all of which is important if you suffer from adrenal fatigue.

Seaweed is rich in minerals and phytonutrients that may be lacking from our regular diet. Many supermarkets have a selection of different seaweeds, and it is a good idea to eat a variety to get the most benefit. This is a quick and easy way to add a nutritional boost to a meal. What you drink can also provide you with many different nutrients and minerals. Fermented drinks are becoming a bit more popular in the American market; they promote good bacteria which helps to improve digestion and nutrient absorption. Two good examples of fermented drinks are kvass and kombucha. Start shopping in different places, check out your local health food stores and farmer's markets. Sometimes specialty items are cheaper, and you can get your standard fruits and vegetables at more traditional grocery stores.

Pay attention to labels, look at the amount of sugar in everything. It is easy to look at something and assume it is healthy when it's full of added sugars. Many additives and preservatives can cause inflammation too, so it is a good idea to stick to fresh or frozen fruits and vegetables over canned items. If you do buy canned products make sure to read the labels too, canned fruit usually has tons of added sugar, and it might not be worth a couple of dollars in savings. Grab circulars and pay attention to sales. Also try new things, having a positive attitude about a lifestyle change will increase your chances of success.

Caffeine Effects

Many people are addicted to a stimulant and take large doses of it every day; they just don't realize it. Caffeine is highly addictive, and many of us consume and crave it in large amounts. It starts off harmless, we drink it when we need an energy boost, and it provides us with it, but it is short-lived. This leads to the up and down energy rollercoaster that coffee so often provides. Each high is shadowed by a low and that low is often followed by a desire to consume more. Many adrenal fatigue sufferers say that their coffee provides less and less energy over time. To make up for this loss, many people start to drink larger cups or combining it with sugary snacks to compensate.

When you drink a cup of coffee, your brain sends a signal to the pituitary gland that releases a hormone which tells your adrenals to create cortisol and adrenaline. In essence, you are creating the same stress response your body would have to stressful situations such as physical danger. This would be fine if you only consume an occasional cup of coffee since they can react capably and quickly to this type of stimulation. However, if you drink several cups of coffee throughout the day you will feel a weakened reaction, some people describe it as their 'tolerance' increasing. The truth is though; your body is not handling it better, your adrenals are weakened and unable to respond appropriately.

The best thing for your adrenal fatigue recovery is giving up caffeine altogether. This may seem like a daunting task, we have all heard of the dreaded caffeine withdrawal symptoms, but the good news is they only last about a week. After quitting coffee, adrenal fatigue sufferers said they have a more consistent, balanced energy level throughout the day.

Some of us just cannot imagine a world without coffee. Much of a coffee addiction is psychological and based on the act of preparation. One thing you can do to make it easier is switching to the decaffeinated version. You still get to go through the actions of making your coffee, and it will taste the same, only without the majority of the potential health risks. Many people rely on caffeine to help us wake up in the morning. Instead of depending on that cup set your alarm half an hour earlier and allow your body to wake up naturally. Room temperature water with a slice of lemon is a good way to encourage the body to function, and quite refreshing too.

Quitting cold turkey means the withdrawal symptoms such as the headaches will come and remind you of your unhealthy addiction. To avoid this reaction, you can try a gradual reduction in caffeine consumption. Once you are ready to give it up completely, do not underestimate your very own will power. When you crave caffeinated drinks, just tell yourself "no, not happening" and move on to a caffeine free alternative. Create a new routine that does not revolve around the preparation or consumption of caffeine. Learn to rely on your natural energy levels and schedule your life around them. Dehydration can also lead to feelings of fatigue, so make sure to drink more water. This is a great way to feel more energized and save money!

Foods that Help Adrenal Function

You have learned about what to avoid, but not much about what to eat to heal from the inside out. Focus on foods that are full of vitamins and minerals. All the B vitamins are important to adrenal function, especially pantothenic acid. The adrenal glands need pantothenic acid to operate smoothly if your body does not have enough the adrenal glands can shrink and become weakened. B vitamins also enhance the activity of the adrenal glands and can increase energy levels during stressful situations. Foods that are high in B vitamins are oats, turkey, beef, Brazil nuts, potatoes, legumes, and bananas.

Another vitamin that adrenal glands depend on when producing cortisol is vitamin C. High levels of vitamin C are stored and used in the adrenal glands, but during the stress response levels of this nutrient seem to drop much quicker than normal. So when you are eating your 8 or 9 servings of fruits and vegetables a day, it is important to include foods that contain high amounts of vitamin C. Common foods high in vitamin C are broccoli, asparagus, Brussel sprouts, spring greens, peaches, tomatoes, citrus fruits, and mangoes.

L-tyrosine is a vitamin that can be found in foods; this vitamin helps to relieve excess stress placed on the adrenal glands. This vitamin also helps the body send signals from one system to another. L-tyrosine levels in the body decline due to stress, so it is important to consume foods rich in this particular vitamin to help the body's healthy stress response. Foods that are high in L-tyrosine are pork, fish, chicken, bananas, whole grains, oats, avocados, seeds, nuts, and legumes.

Now that you know what vitamins and foods help to heal you from the inside out, it is up to you to incorporate them into your diet. It is not necessary to only eat the foods on the list since all vegetables and fruits are good for your health, you just now have a better understanding of which ones to focus on. You can mix them into your normal dinners or make special vitamin-rich smoothies or meals that are made only of adrenal improving foods.

Supplements

Not only does adrenal fatigue cause a hormone deficiency, but your body could also be short on many of the vitamins, nutrients, and compounds it needs to operate efficiently. Your blood tests might have shown levels that fall within the reference range, but as you know, that is not always the best way to determining factor. Similar to the hormones, you should be focusing on maintaining the optimal level of these vitamins and nutrients and not just the minimum. Herbs and probiotics can also help you recover from adrenal fatigue faster by helping your body absorb nutrients and maintain energy levels. Finding the right combination for you is important, so it is essential to listen to your body. Just like everyone doesn't suffer from the same set of symptoms, not everyone needs to be on the same set of supplements. There is no one size fits all when it comes to adrenal recovery and what works for one person might not work for another. When purchasing your herbs, supplements, and probiotics make sure you get high-quality products and try to buy only organic if possible.

Vitamins B5, B6, B12 are often lacking in adrenal fatigue sufferers and are easy to replace using supplements. These vitamins play an important role in improving metabolic pathways which increase energy levels and reduces fatigue. Vitamin B4 plays a part in the creation of coenzyme A, which aids in cellular respiration and the breakdown of carbohydrates, fats, and proteins. Vitamin B6 is involved in several of the pathways that are used to create adrenal hormones. Vitamin B12 supports cell repair, energy production, and the maintenance of red blood cells. Many supplements on the market combine all three into one pill, so it is easy and convenient.

Vitamin C supplements are often recommended since so many of us do not get enough of the vitamin from the foods we eat. In addition to being a powerful antioxidant vitamin C is also directly involved in cortisol production. This particular vitamin is essential in the recovery of our adrenal glands. Begin by taking 1000 mg and then gradually increasing your dose; it should be taken with bioflavonoids, similar to how it occurs in nature.

It is estimated that 75% of Americans suffer from a Magnesium deficiency. Magnesium helps our body control our energy flow, which is important when trying to get back to healthy and normal energy levels. The symptoms of a Magnesium deficiency can be fatigue, depression, insomnia, cramping, and muscle stiffness. Taking too much

Magnesium can cause digestive issues so be careful with your starting dose, 400 mg is a safe introduction.

The health benefits of probiotics have a wealth of scientific studies backing them up. Among other things, they can help reduce stress levels, improve digestion, and reduce the side-effects of antibiotics. When we improve our digestion, we are increasing the number of nutrients our body can absorb from the foods we eat. In turn, we are helping our body heal itself by providing a foundation of essential vitamins and minerals that it needs to maintain energy levels and produce the hormones we need. Probiotics also help to strengthen our immune system which can help ward off illness and prevent our adrenal glands from becoming even more overworked. Look for a probiotic that has at least 10 billion colony forming units and five different strains of bacteria.

Herbs have been used for centuries in traditional cultures for medicinal purposes, and they can play an important role in overcoming adrenal fatigue. They can be taken in conjunction with other supplements and can aid in your recovery. It is important to note, that you do not have to take everything on the list, only take what you need.

Licorice Root

This root is used to increase endurance, stimulate hormone production, and maintain energy levels. This is a great choice for adrenal fatigue sufferers because it helps cortisol circulate for longer periods of time. However, it can raise your blood pressure. If you are one of the rare individuals that have high blood pressure and adrenal fatigue, this herb might not be ideal for you.

Ashwagandha

This is known an adaptogenic herb that helps to regulate many different systems within the body. For instance, if cortisol is too high it helps to lower it, and if it is too low, it helps to raise it.

Siberian Ginseng

Russian Olympic athletes use this herb to increase their stamina. However, it can also be used to boost energy levels and improve mental awareness. Just like licorice root, though, it can also increase blood pressure, so it is not meant for everyone.

Maca Root

Studies show that this herb can positively affect cortisol regulation and blood sugar. It also allows for more effective uptake of hormones into cells, thus increasing their efficiency. If you suffer from adrenal fatigue and have lower than normal hormone levels, you can take Maca root to make the most of the hormones you do have.

Omega-3

Many of us do not have optimal amounts of Omega-3 fatty acids from the foods we eat, but we do tend to have an adequate amount of Omega-6. This creates an imbalance that can lead to inflammation that requires cortisol production to manage. Taking Omega-3 can reduce the workload placed on your adrenals by reducing inflammation throughout the body.

It is important to read labels for recommended dosage on all supplements and herbs. Many supplements behave differently within the body depending on the dose, so you want to make sure you are helping yourself get better and not worse. The exact dose of some supplements is not well-known or established, so it is important to listen to your body and tweak your dosage appropriately. So just take your time when deciding which supplements and herbs are right for you. There is not one correct formula that rids you of adrenal fatigue. It is a process that can take months, these supplements are meant to make this journey easier and faster, but are by no means a cure-all.

Chapter 5: Lifestyle Changes that Accelerate Recovery

The power of the mind over the body is often overlooked in modern medicine. In recent years psychological changes have been found to have a real impact on our physical health. Stress is a great example of this because stress is a mental state that has the power to trigger many different physical changes within our bodies. These changes can impact nearly all the organs and systems that are vital to our good health. Prolonged exposure to stress can lead to chronic illness such as adrenal fatigue. It is with this in mind that one of the ways to improve chronic fatigue syndrome is to address the main causes of stress in our lives. Similar to the way that our mental health can cause physical problems, it assumed that improving our emotional well-being can help to reverse these disorders.

Exercise

Depending on which stage of adrenal fatigue you are in will determine what types of exercise you can do safely. If you are in the last two stages, your adrenal glands cannot produce the hormones needed for more vigorous activities such as going for a run or soccer, because after the temporary high is over it will inevitably result in an adrenal crash. Such exercises like swimming, yoga, or walking are better because they are low-impact. However, if you are in the first two stages, then you can lift weights and go for a run because exercise tends to help regulate cortisol levels.

Get your exercise routine in early in the day, waiting too long can disrupt our natural sleep cycles. If you get it out the way early, you also reap the added benefit of a metabolism boost. People who are older find that long periods of exercise drain too much of their energy, but younger people can exercise for longer periods of time. So be careful not to overexert yourself to the point of exhaustion.

Deep Breathing and Meditation

Studies show that meditation can change our circulatory patterns, brain waves, and immune response. That is pretty impressive considering most of the medical world forgets about the power of the mind over the body. Meditation and deep breathing can be beneficial at all four stages. If you are in the first two stages, it can help you reduce stress and stabilize adrenaline and cortisol levels. If you are in the last two stages, it can help you improve circulation and increase energy levels.

Meditation sounds difficult; it is often very hard for us to sit still for two minutes, making 15 or 20 minutes seem nearly impossible. However, there is a long list of reasons to do it, so find a nice quiet area and settle in for at least 15 minutes. It is not necessary to force yourself into the lotus position if you are comfortable that way, you can sit on the floor with your hands on your lap, or you can even sit in a chair if you prefer, just make sure to maintain the natural curve of your back. Gently close your eyes and begin by taking slow, deep breaths, inhaling through your nose and exhaling through your mouth. Your first few breaths will most likely be shallow, but as you continue to breathe, they will become full and deep. Focus on each breath you take, be aware of the air entering and exiting your lungs. If you find your attention straying simply bring it back by letting thoughts simply float by, do not get frustrated just continue to focus on your breathing. Just like with other things, practice makes perfect and the more you meditate, the easier it will be to maintain focus. When it is time to end your session open your eyes and slowly stand up. Repeat this once or twice a day.

Stress Reduction

There are some things you can do to help yourself deal with stress. A great way to prevent the impact stressors have on you is to prep or prepare for them. For example, if you know you have a business meeting, make sure you have everything ready. You can even lay out your clothes and make a breakfast that will keep overnight, so you will have more time to collect yourself beforehand.

Listening to meditative or soft music helps to alleviate stress. The perfect time for a quick listen is during a drive or on your ride to work. Add some muscle relaxation to this for even more stress relief. Simply grab your steering wheel and clench the muscles in your back, arms, shoulders, and fingers until they tremble, hold this for 45 seconds and then release. This will cause a wave of relief to spread throughout your upper body, be careful not to let your hands off the steering wheel!

A Swedish study found that floating in water can trigger the body's relaxation response, which helps lower stress hormone levels. This is not going to be true for people who are uneasy in the water. If you are not truly comfortable in the water, then do not attempt this because you run the risk of it increasing your stress levels. Choose your pool of water based on your preferences and limitations.

Learning to worry about one thing a time can go a long way in helping you cope with stress in a more healthy way. Doing this keeps you from feeling the overwhelming and crushing feeling of having multiple problems looming over you. Learn to tell the difference between real-life problems and tune out imagined ones. The brain cannot tell the difference between a real and perceived threat, so imagined stressors can have just as much of an impact of a real stressor.

Talk or write about what is bothering you. If you have a group of friends or family members that you feel comfortable talking to, set up a time to meet with them. If that is not an option, writing in a journal or even a computer screen is enough to make you feel less alone.

Learn to speak a stress-free language, people who handle stress well have a tendency to use what stress experts call an "optimistic explanatory style." They do not dwell on things that don't work out in their favor, and instead of making negative enveloping statements, they would focus on one thing they could do better. Instead of saying you "expect" something, retrain yourself to say "hope" instead.

Laughter improves immune function and relieves tension, but one of the fastest ways to kill a sense of humor is anxiety and stress. With that logic, it would also mean that it is almost impossible to feel stressed when you are in the middle of a giggling fit. So watch that comedy that never fails to make you laugh or hang out with your funniest friend. Anything to make the genuine laughs come.

Attempt the impossible and pick out one good thing that happened each and every day and think about it. This is a common scenario for many of us: coming home and immediately venting to our spouse or roommate about what an awful day it's been. Next time, instead of creating a negative atmosphere, lead with the positive.

No matter how much you don't want to, don't skip your workout routine. Make sure you stick to your schedule and don't start skipping workouts because it can become a habit. Exercise is one of the best ways to help release stress, but you can only reap this benefit if you do it.

Having a positive and open mind is one your best weapons against adrenal fatigue. As you have learned the power of the mind over the body can be powerful, and the same is true for attitude. You are more likely to succeed if you think you can and you are open to making the changes. If you go into it with a negative outlook you will only cause yourself more stress, slowing your progress and your recovery. Try not to beat yourself up over your mistakes, instead, correct your behavior and continue to move on.

You can do one relaxation or stress relieving technique or combine a few of them to find what works for you. Meditation is recommended for all sufferers of adrenal fatigue since it has so many benefits, but how you do it is personal preference. Everyone who suffers from adrenal fatigue wishes there was a simple cure that happened fast, but in reality, recovery takes a lot of work and can take anywhere from 6 to 18 months. However, once you start to make some progress, you will feel energized and want to keep making these positive changes. Just keep working towards your goal and doing the stress reduction techniques that work for you, and before you know it, you will be well on your way to a full recovery.

Recovery depends on many different factors such as the severity of the adrenal fatigue and your willingness to make the necessary lifestyle changes. The more severe the adrenal fatigue, the longer it is going to take to recover. The more the body has to recover from the time it needs to recuperate. You are probably going to try to rush it, but take joy in the little things that make it easier. Learn to celebrate the small breakthroughs instead of focusing on the big picture. Smaller goals are easier and faster to achieve, and they add up to much larger goals. The path to recovery can be difficult, but with patience and hard work you can get there.

Conclusion

Thank you again for downloading this book!

I hope this book was able to help you to help you choose your path for adrenal fatigue recovery. The next step is to make the changes needed to ensure a full recovery.

Thank you and good luck!

www.ingramcontent.com/pod-product-compliance
Lightning Source LLC
Chambersburg PA
CBHW070402190526
45169CB00003B/1074